PELVIC FLOOR WELLNESS FOR SENIORS

EASY EXERCISES TO COMBAT DYSFUNCTION

LUNA WELLNESS

LEGAL NOTICE

DISCLAIMER NOTICE

Please note the information contained within this document is for educational and entertainment purposes only. All effort has been executed to present accurate, up to date, reliable, complete information. No warranties of any kind are declared or implied. Readers acknowledge that the author is not engaged in the rendering of legal, financial, medical or professional advice. The content within this book has been derived from various sources. Please consult a licensed professional before attempting any techniques outlined in this book.

By reading this document, the reader agrees that under no circumstances is the author responsible for any losses, direct or indirect, that are incurred as a result of the use of the information contained within this document, including, but not limited to, errors, omissions, or inaccuracies.

TABLE OF CONTENTS

To learn more about vibrant living and to get 5 bonus exercises visit our website at:

fitness.luna-wellness.net/5cbc473d

SCAN ME

INTRODUCTION

Welcome to "Pelvic Floor Wellness for Seniors: Easy Exercises to Combat Dysfunction, Achieve Continence, and Revitalize Sexual Health." This book is designed with one goal in mind: to help you, the reader, understand the importance of pelvic floor health, especially as it pertains to the unique challenges faced by seniors, and to provide you with the knowledge and tools you need to improve or maintain it from the comfort of your home.

The pelvic floor is a key set of muscles that lie at the base of the pelvis. These muscles play a crucial role in supporting your pelvic organs, contributing to urinary and fecal continence, and enhancing sexual function. Despite their importance, the pelvic floor is often overlooked in general fitness routines, particularly for the senior population. As we age, the muscles in our pelvic floor can weaken due to various factors such as surgery, childbirth, heavy lifting, chronic coughing, or simply the natural aging process. This weakening can lead to several uncomfortable or even debilitating conditions, including incontinence, pelvic organ prolapse, pelvic pain, and sexual dysfunction.

Understanding these issues is the first step towards empowerment. This book is designed to be a comprehensive guide that will walk you through the anatomy of the pelvic floor, explain its functions, and outline common pelvic floor disorders that seniors face. More importantly, it will introduce you to a series of easy-to-follow exercises and lifestyle changes that can help strengthen the pelvic floor, alleviate symptoms associated with its dysfunction, and improve your overall quality of life.

We have structured this book to be as informative and accessible as possible. Whether you are a senior experiencing pelvic floor issues, a caregiver, or simply someone interested in maintaining your pelvic health as you age, this book is for you. We begin by laying the foundation with essential background information on the pelvic floor, then progress to practical exercise routines that can be tailored to fit individual needs and abilities. Along the way, we provide safety tips, address common challenges, and offer advice on integrating these practices into your daily life for lasting benefits.

Our hope is that by the end of this book, you will not only have gained a deeper understanding of your pelvic floor and how to care for it but also feel equipped and motivated to incorporate these exercises into your routine. Remember, it's never too late to start focusing on your pelvic health. By taking small steps today, you can improve your wellbeing, boost your confidence, and enjoy a more active, fulfilling life.

Let's embark on this journey together, with patience, persistence, and positivity. Welcome to a stronger, healthier you.

CHAPTER 1: UNDERSTANDING THE PELVIC FLOOR

Although we have heard about the pelvic floor quite a few times, do we have an anatomical understanding of what a pelvic floor is, and what it does to the human body?

This chapter breaks down the basic functions of a pelvic floor, and how pelvic floor muscles equip the human body to perform some cardinal functions.

Anatomy of the Pelvic Floor

Most of you would be familiar with the pelvic region of the human body. Many important organs of our body, including the urinary bladder, bowels, and reproductive organs, are situated in the region, which is, in turn, supported by the pelvic floor. In simple terms, it is made up of muscles and connective tissues, which form a supportive bed, which not only protects these organs, but helps us stabilize our bodies while performing functions like urinating, defecting, or doing sexual activity. In other words, the twin cardinal functions of the pelvic floor include protecting the vital pelvic organs from external damage or shock, maintaining the core, and helping us have control over bodily functions.

In females, the pelvic floor not only helps in defecating and urinating, but also regulates vaginal contractions, and plays an important role during vaginal childbirth. In males, the pelvic floor contains the prostate in addition to the urethra, bowel, rectum, and anus, thus assisting in the process of ejaculation and erection of the sexual organ, in addition to defecating and urinating.

The muscles of the pelvic floor are divided into two, commonly known as levator ani and coccygeus muscles. The former category is subdivided into two, referred to as pubococcygeus muscles, which form the inner layer, and iliococcygeus muscles, which form the outer layer. Levator ani constitutes the greater part of the pelvic floor, thus rendering the functions of supporting the pelvic floor, and protection of its organs. Coccygeus muscles play an important role in the expansion and contraction of the coccyx and urethra, thus supporting the functions of defecation and urination.

Functions of the Pelvic Floor Muscles

The pelvic floor muscles play multiple roles when it comes to our physiological functions. Some of them are:

1. Supportive Function- As we know, the human pelvis is shaped in a particular way, which is designed to protect the internal pelvic organs, and provide stability to our body. In addition to the skeletal structure, pelvic muscles also play an integral role in the support of the structure of the pelvis, as well as protection of the pelvic organs.

2. The function of the sphincters- Sphincters are bands of muscles that surround pelvic organs like the urethra, anus, vagina, or prostate. The contraction and release of pelvic floor muscles are the regulators of the sphincters, which consequentially tighten or release the openings of these organs. For example, when the pelvic floor muscles are contracted, the sphincters tighten, thus contracting the openings of these organs. When the pelvic floor muscles are released, the sphincters are also released, which help in defecation and urination.

3. Sexual Function: In both men and women, pelvic floor muscles play an important role in sexual performance. In men, expansion and contraction of pelvic floor muscles are what results in erection of the male sexual organ, as well as ejaculation. In women, contraction of the pelvic floor muscles helps in sexual arousal.

4. The function of Stability: Although we have heard about stabilizing the core and the need to keep our core straight, have we thought about what exactly constitutes our body's core? Well, think of it like this. Imagine our body as a line, and the central point is constituted by the core. It consists

of our abdominal muscles, sometimes referred to as abs, muscles of the lower back region, hips, and pelvic floor muscles. Along with the other muscles, the pelvic floor muscles help in keeping our body erect and stabilized. It supports the spine, thereby performing one of the most integral functions in our body.

Common Pelvic Floor Disorders in Seniors

As we age, like all other muscles and tissues, pelvic floor muscles will also undergo wear and tear, thus resulting in some disorders, out of which the common ones are:

1. Pelvic Organ prolapse: As the term suggests, this is a condition that affects the organs situated in the pelvic region, where one or more organs could drop from their original position, thus creating pain or discomfort. This is resulted from the pelvic floor muscles getting loose.

2. Incontinence: As the pelvic floor muscles get weakened, their ability to regulate the functions of urination and defection will also get affected, thus resulting in incontinence, or loss of regulatory abilities of urinary and bowel functions. Among seniors, three types of incontinence are most commonly found, which are stress incontinence, urge incontinence, and mixed incontinence. The first is perhaps the most common one, which is experienced whenever one puts a pressure on the bladder either by sneezing, coughing, or lifting weights. On the other hand, urge incontinence is characterized by frequent urges to urinate, which is followed by a sudden release of urine, which is often uncontrollable due to the weakened pelvic floor muscles. This is a reason why seniors experience the urge for more frequent bathroom breaks, which could affect the quality of their lives. Some people could also experience a combination of stress incontinence and urge incontinence, which is referred to as mixed incontinence.

3. Pain: Seniors are more prone to experiencing pain around the pelvic area, which could have several reasons. In women, it could be an underlying

cause of ovarian abnormalities, including endometriosis or fibroids. However, tension in pelvic floor muscles is an important cause of pelvic pain. In some cases, it could be accompanied by symptoms like constipation, irritable bowel syndrome, or pain while urinating, defecating, or during intercourse. This could be a collective symptom of pelvic floor dysfunction, which is the inability to use the muscles of the pelvic floor, which is caused by multiple factors, including injury and aging.

4. Sexual Dysfunction: As mentioned before, weakened pelvic floor muscles could create painful sexual intercourse in women, thus affecting the quality of sexual experience. Similarly, in men, it could create erectile dysfunction and an inability to ejaculate, as those functions are primarily controlled by the pelvic floor muscles.

Factors Contributing to Pelvic Floor Issues in Seniors

Although muscular wear and tear due to ageing is a primary factor when it comes to pelvic floor dysfunction, there are other factors could exacerbate the issue.

1. Ageing- Naturally, as one ages, the muscular and skeletal tissues go through wear and tear, thus impacting its functions.

2. Surgical Procedures: Surgeries done in the pelvic area, be it prostatectomy or hysterectomy, could affect the function of pelvic floor muscles. In fact, research shows that those individuals who have undergone hysterectomy are at a higher risk for pelvic organ prolapse and urinary incontinence(Forsgren et al., 2022).

3. Childbirth: In women, pregnancy and associated childbirth could affect the pelvic floor muscles. Especially during the later phase of pregnancy, the fetus moves down into the pelvic area, which could cause the muscles to stretch. This impacts the elastic nature of the muscles, which is the reason why many women experience frequent urination and incontinence during the later phase of their pregnancy. Vaginal delivery could also create minor wear and tear in the pelvic muscles(Callewaert et al., 2015).

4. Lifestyle: Some lifestyle factors could make you more prone to pelvic floor dysfunction than others. For example, research shows that individuals with chronic cough tend to exert more pressure on their pelvic floor, thus rendering themselves more prone to pelvic floor dysfunction. Similarly, high-impact exercises such as abdominal crunches or sit-ups, or lifting heavy weights could be detrimental to your pelvic floor if overdone. If you are someone with chronic constipation and regularly exert pressure to relieve yourselves, you might be at a greater risk for pelvic floor dysfunction. Obesity is another lifestyle factor that makes us prone to weakened pelvic muscles.

5. Hormonal Changes: In women, menopause is a hormonal change that results in lowered levels of estrogen and progesterone, which reduces the elasticity of pelvic floor muscles. Similarly, the male hormone testosterone is proven to have a positive effect in the building of muscle tissues. A decline in the levels of this hormone could result in weakened pelvic floor muscles.

CHAPTER 2: THE IMPORTANCE OF PELVIC FLOOR EXERCISES

Benefits of Strengthening the Pelvic Floor

- Improved Bladder and Bowel Control:

Martin has almost retired from partaking in the major joys of his life, which includes hiking and other outdoor adventures, citing that he has almost reached the latter half of sixties. His friends often make fun of him and his adopted grandfather mode, but they do not realise the major reason of his withdrawal, which happens to be the 'unexpected cases of leaking', which makes him dread going out.

Does this sound like a familiar scenario? Urinary and bowel incontinence are more common than we think they are, which is due to the fact that we do not attach much importance to practicing pelvic floor strengthening exercises. The good news is that, it is not too late for Martin, for regular pelvic floor exercises can strengthen the muscles, thus improving the condition of incontinence, and thereby improving the quality of his life.

- Support for Pelvic Organ Prolapse:

Pelvic organ prolapse happens when one or more pelvic organs move down from their position, due to loose pelvic muscles. Although this could be uncomfortable and painful, this is also reversible in many cases, especially if it is diagnosed in the earlier stages. Research shows that pelvic floor exercises are the best remedies for reversal of organ prolapse(Hagen et al., 2014), without the need for surgical intervention.

- Enhanced Sexual Function:

Many of us believe that people cease to be sexually active in their senior years. However, this is a huge misconception as people do experience the need for intimacy in their older years, although there could be physical roadblocks to the same, which include a weakened pelvic floor. A weakened pelvic floor could create sexual dissatisfaction, as it might lead to painful sex in females, as well as erectile dysfunction in males. Regular pelvic floor exercises make the muscles stronger, thereby preventing such issues.

- Increased core Stability and Balance

As we age, we might find ourselves in a precarious situation, as far as balance is concerned. This is a reason why older people are more prone to losing their balance, and falling down, which could lead to potential injuries. Our pelvic floor, along with abdominal and hip muscles, play a significant role in maintaining the balance of the body. Stronger pelvic floor measles lend us a stronger core and improved stability.

Impact on Incontinence

Incontinence or loss of control over one's bladder and bowels is often a problem that leads to diminished self-confidence, which adversely impacts the quality of our lives. This could lead people to limit their social interactions, and thus plunge themselves into loneliness.

While some people might feel a sudden urge to urinate, but tends to urinate before they find a toilet, some others could find themselves 'leaking' while sneezing or coughing. The former, known as urge incontinence, and the latter, known as stress incontinence, are commonly experienced by seniors, due to weakened pelvic floor muscles. In both these cases, pelvic floor exercises are remedial in nature, and it will improve the quality of our lives.

Overall Health and Improvement in Quality of Life

Other than drastic improvements in physical health, regular practice of pelvic floor exercises is also beneficial in imparting psychological benefits to our lives.

As we advance into the senior years of our lives, we naturally long for intimacy and human contact, which needs social settings and relationships. However, many people find it difficult to expose themselves in such settings, in fear of embracing themselves due to incontinence. Research shows that urinary incontinence is found in almost 45% of the senior population, which is a testimony of the gravity of the condition(Batmani et al., 2021). Prevention and even reversal of incontinence is possible, through regular practice of pelvic floor exercises, which could help the senior population find renewed self-esteem, and purpose in life.

Moreover, the physical benefits of pelvic floor exercises go beyond prevention of incontinence. Since pelvic floor muscles are also responsible for fortifying the core and stability of the body, stronger pelvic muscles help us develop better posture, thus preventing the possibility of back pain.

Let us look at the example of Mr. Jeff Philips, who has always looked forward to his retirement, to enjoy life to the fullest, with his grandchildren and the rest of his family. However, occasional back pain interfered with his jolly sessions with his grandchildren, and he was soon reduced to the grumpy grandpa who was always complaining about the uncomfortable furniture. A person who used to love to go for evening walks, he soon found himself losing balance easily, and stopped going for walks altogether, in the fear of falling down and embracing himself. Fortunately, he was paid a visit by his childhood friend Arthur, who listened to his friend's complaints, with empathy. Arthur soon shared his secret to a healthy and happy post-retirement life, his regular pelvic floor exercise routine. It did not take much to convince Philips, who was able to transform himself into who he imagined to be, the loving and wonderful grandpa, who was always down for a game!

Establishing a Routine

Before starting an exercise routine, we need to be mindful of a few points. Age and time are important factors when it comes to exercise. Exercising is not a one-size-fits-all program, but should be tailored according to individual preferences and requirements. Each of us are different, and we possibly might have different health conditions, and other criteria. Before integrating pelvic floor exercises into our daily routine, we must be careful not to overwhelm ourselves with difficult techniques. Start slow, and remember that what matters in the long run is consistency, and not the complexity.

Setting goals will help us to stay motivated and will also help us in tracking progress, but the goals need to be realistic and rooted. If you set overly ambitious goals, it is possible for you to either overexert yourself or be demotivated soon. To avoid this from happening, we need to set our goals based on our individual health conditions and time, thus prioritising progress over perfection.

To ensure that our exercise routine is sustainable and productive, we need to make sure to avoid overexertion. By being mindful while exercising, one can spot the signs of overexertion, and thus avoid further complications. Signs like having a very high pulse rate, experiencing abdominal pain, sweating vigorously, or feeling dizzy are some common symptoms of overexertion. If you feel any of these symptoms, take a break, hydrate yourselves, and bring the complexity of the exercise down a few notches. For the same reason, it is advised to seek the help of a trained professional, who will be able to guide you according to your specific needs, as opposed to general videos that are not intended for a niche category.

CHAPTER 3: PREPARING FOR PELVIC FLOOR EXERCISES

While it could be easy to follow a number of steps intended for a wide demography, this book intends to bring a difference, by catering for a specific group. Read on, to discover the basic tenets of preparing for a pelvic floor exercise regimen.

How to Identify Your Pelvic Floor Muscles

The first step before starting the exercise regimen is to identify your pelvic floor muscles. Training the muscles of your biceps or abdomen is easier, as we are more or less aware about their precise location. How do we find the precise location of our pelvic floor muscles? One of the most widely used techniques is to imagine resisting the passing of wind. For example, if you are in a crowd or out on a date, but you feel as if you are about to pass the wind, chances are that you would try to resist it. Now, imagine the sensation. the muscles that we employ in the action of resisting the passage of wind are the pelvic floor muscles. Similarly, when you are in the process of urinating, and if you try to temporarily stop the process, you will be squeezing the pelvic floor muscles.

However, if you are a woman, the muscles that you employ to squeeze your vagina are the pelvic floor muscles. On the contrary, if you are a man, the muscles that you employ when you try to move your penis without moving any other part of the body, would be the pelvic floor muscles.

Since we cannot see the pelvic floor muscles in action, few visualization techniques could be used while exercising, which many people find useful. While exercising, you will have to switch on and off your pelvic muscles, which could be a difficult feat initially but can be easily achieved through visualization. For example, imagine a pebble falling into the water. There will be ringlets of water formed around the pebble, and water rising around it. In other words, the ringlets of water are drawing close to the central point of the fall, which is similar to the pelvic floor which is lifting and rising above its neutral position. Now, imagine the same visual, but with the ringlets of water departing away from the central point. This is your off position, where the pelvic floor falls.

Breathwork and Its Role in Pelvic Floor Exercises

While breath work is important in all kinds of exercises, it plays a cardinal role in pelvic floor workouts.

Let us consider the role of diaphragm muscles and pelvic floor muscles in breathing. As we know, our breathing is composed of inhalation, when we take air in, and exhalation, when we push air out. During inhalation, the diaphragm muscles and the pelvic floor muscles move downwards. While exhalation, the diaphragm muscles move upwards, while the pelvic floor muscles resume their original position, again moving upwards. This movement occurs in tandem, which helps us in seamless breathing.

For the pelvic floor muscles to be properly engaged during the exercise, and for them to relax post-exercise, one needs to be mindful of proper breathwork techniques. Although there are a number of breathing techniques, nothing comes close to diaphragmatic breathing, when it comes to enhancing the strength of the pelvic floor. While we normally breathe in and out through the nose, diaphragmatic breathing is slightly different. Take a deep inhalation through the nose. You will notice that the diaphragm has expanded during the inhalation. Next, exhale sharply through the mouth. You will notice your pelvic floor muscles relaxing during the exhalation. In addition to reducing blood pressure, this also has the additional benefit of imparting more relaxation to your entire body.

If you are looking for a more relaxed breathing exercise, you could try belly breathing. Lie down on your back, and place your head on a pillow. Make sure you are lying down in a comfortable position. Place a hand on your chest, and place the other hand on your abdomen. Take a deep inhalation through the nose, where you can feel the diaphragm expanding. Hold your breath for a couple of seconds, and exhale through the mouth. You will feel the pelvic muscles relaxing.

Establishing a Routine: Best Times for Exercise

The best time for exercise is whenever you have time. However, most of us might find it difficult to set aside organized time slots for exercise, given how busy our schedules could be. Although it is always best to be consistent with our exercise schedule, it is not only clever, but also productive to combine the exercise routine with other habitual activities. For example, you might have seen people listening to important podcasts or audiobooks while running or lifting weights. Similarly, you can integrate your pelvic floor exercises into your daily routine, be it while watching TV, brushing your teeth, or even cooking or doing daily chores.

However, pelvic floor exercises yield the best results when the body is relaxed and composed. This is why most pelvic floor exercises are done while you remain seated or in a comfortable position. It is crucial therefore to listen to your body before attempting to do pelvic floor exercises.

Mindful Engagement with Pelvic Floor Health

Mindfulness is a keyword we have been hearing quite often, in recent times. However, mindfulness is far from a novel concept, as it has been practiced by Buddhist monks and ascetics in history. This simple concept involves being more aware of ourselves, or utilizing our senses in whatever we are doing. B eat listening to your body and your surroundings, being acutely aware of the sights, smells, and textures around you, mindfulness helps us stay focused and live in the present. It is important to be mindful while doing pelvic floor exercises, as it enhances focus, and effectiveness, and helps in recognizing the body's responses. Mindfulness also helps us actively listen to our body, and set reasonable goals according to our bodily requirements.

CHAPTER 4: BASIC PELVIC FLOOR EXERCISES

Now that we are past the preparation phase, let us proceed to familiarising ourselves with the fundamentals of pelvic floor exercises.

Although these are simple and basic enough for a beginner to attempt, these exercises form the core of a pelvic strengthening routine, as these are effective and sustainable enough to yield long-term results. These do not require any equipment, and could be done in the comfort of your homes.

Kegel Exercises: Technique and Variations

Kegel exercises are specially designed to strengthen the pelvic floor muscles, and are particularly effective against incontinence and pelvic floor dysfunction. One of the major advantages of a Kegel routine is that it is simple enough to do anywhere, at any time, which gives us much room for customization and personalization.

Before doing the Kegel exercise, ensure that you have determined the correct location of your pelvic floor muscles, using any of the techniques mentioned in the previous chapter. You can do kegels in any position, whether standing, sitting, or lying down. If doing it for the first time, try doing it lying down, as it helps you in relaxing the body. Imagine that you are sitting on top of a small ball. Try to lift the ball without using your limbs, by squeezing the pelvic floor muscles. Squeeze for a couple of seconds, and then relax. Repeat four to five times.

A few mistakes a beginner could make while doing Kegel exercises are as follows. One might apply so much pressure into doing Kegels, that they might hold their breath. This could be contrary to the expected outcome, as you are supposed to breathe freely and deeply while doing the exercise. Secondly, only the pelvic floor muscles need to be occupied while doing the exercise. Beginners could also be employing the abdominal muscles or the leg muscles, which should be kept in a relaxed state.

There are many variations to performing Kegel exercises. The 4-3-2 method is a popular one, in which four sets of Kegel exercises are done, each set containing three squeezes each. Make sure you are giving ample time for contraction as well as relaxation of the muscles. For example, one set of Kegel exercises will contain three contractions and three relaxations. Each contraction should be of two breaths, followed by two breaths of relaxation. Remember that proper relaxation of pelvic floor muscles is equally important. Depending on the time taken to hold the contractions, Kegel exercises are divided into quick muscle contractions and long-hold muscle contractions. As a beginner, you could rely on quick muscle contractions, lasting for a couple of seconds, and slowly proceed to long-hold muscle contractions.

KEGEL EXERCISES

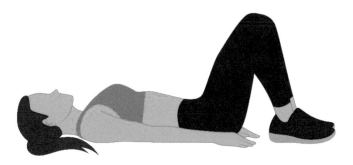

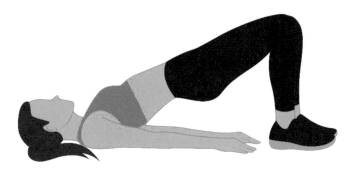

- Identify the pelvic floor muscles by trying to stop your urine mid-stream. These are the muscles you need to activate.
- Empty your bladder and lie down or sit comfortably.
- Contract the pelvic floor muscles for a count of three to five seconds.
- Relax for a count of three to five seconds.
- Repeat 10 to 15 times per session, and aim for three sessions per day.

Bridging for Pelvic Floor Strength

Bridges are quite effective for enhancing the strength of pelvic floor muscles. One of the chief advantages of bridges is that the exercise is not only good for the pelvic floor, but also effective for the glutes and hamstrings.

Lie on your back on a yoga mat, in a comfortable position. Your knees should be bent at the right angle, while your arms can rest along your sides, with their palms facing down. Ensure that your back is straight, and lies flat against the ground. Your feet should be resting flat on the ground. Push with your heels, and slowly raise your hips, while squeezing the muscles of the glutes, hamstrings, and pelvic floor. A common mistake many people make while doing bridges is to push yourself up using the lower back muscles, which could be quite detrimental to your lower back muscles, leading to injury. Hence, be mindful, and push using the heels, and consciously raise the hip. Hold the position for a couple of seconds, and resume to the original position.

A variation of the regular bridge pose is an elevated bridge pose, where you could choose to rest your feet on an exercise ball, which is easier than the normal bridge position. Those individuals with back pain should be careful while doing bridges, and could use a support to rest their sacrum, in order to avoid exacerbating their symptoms.

BRIDGING

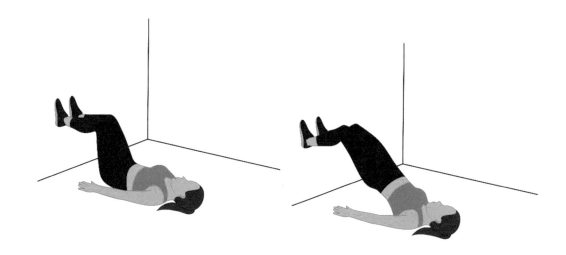

- Lie on your back with your knees bent and feet flat on the floor, hip-width apart.
- Press your feet into the floor, inhale, and lift your hips off the floor towards the ceiling.
- Pause at the top for a few seconds, then exhale and slowly lower your hips back to the floor.
- Do 10 to 15 repetitions.

Seated Exercises for Pelvic Engagement

For those who have difficulty in doing exercises while standing, seated pelvic floor exercises come in handy. This is also effective for those who spend a major part of their day sitting, as the exercise not only relieves monotony, but also enhances the pelvic floor muscles.

Make sure that you are seated on a comfortable chair with back support. Do not slump your shoulders, but sit in an erect manner, with your feet comfortably planted on the floor. Take a deep breath. While exhaling, squeeze your pelvic floor muscles, in the same way as if you are trying to stop yourself from urinating. Hold the squeeze for a couple of seconds, but remember not to hold your breath. Rest, and take a deep inhalation, followed by exhalation. Repeat the process for three to four times. If you face any difficulties, try employing visualization techniques or even saying 'shhhh...' while exhaling could be beneficial in relaxing and finding the right muscles. Let us look at some powerful visualization techniques.

Visualization Techniques to Enhance Effectiveness

Very often, when we do an exercise for the first time, we could experience difficulty in focusing. This could be due to a number of factors, including anxiety. To prevent this from happening, visualisation techniques could be used. For example, let us look at how Peter performs seated pelvic squeezes.

Peter has seated himself comfortably, and has taken a deep inhalation. While exhaling, he squeezes his pelvic floor muscles, while he imagines his office lift going up. He conjures up the vision with rich imagery. The lift with its gleaming silver surface, the red knobs on which different numbers are plastered with green letters. Other than him, there are two other people in the lift, who are getting down at the third and fourth floors. Numbers gleam on the digital surface, while the lift slowly goes up. He can smell the cologne of his neighbor, and he wishes them good morning.

Such an effective imagery will help us stay focused, and relaxes ourselves, without our knowledge. You could also imagine a peaceful seashore or a garden, with all the sensory details.

Incorporating Exercises into Daily Life

Basic pelvic floor exercises are flexible and simple enough to be incorporated into your daily life. If you are able to set aside a fixed time slot for regular exercise, well and good! However, not all of us might be able to afford the luxury of time, and for such individuals, incorporating pelvic floor exercises into your daily life is a good alternative. For example, let us start from the beginning of the day. Pelvic squeezes could be done while brushing your teeth or getting ready for the day. Seated squeezes could be done while watching the news or even between your daily work. If you are able to snatch ten minutes between your work, set it aside for a session of kegels or bridges.

Lifestyle adjustments are also required for enhanced pelvic floor muscles. This might begin with the way you sleep, for example. Sleeping on one's stomach is not ideal for enhanced pelvic floor muscles, and could lead to a weakened pelvic floor in the long run. By changing the position of your sleep, you can avoid that pitfall. Ensure that your posture is conducive to good pelvic floor health. For instance, avoid slouching, and pay particular attention while lifting heavy objects or doing abdominal exercises. When it comes to your diet, limit the intake of caffeine, sugar, carbonated drinks, and spicy foods, but increase the intake of vitamin C, vitamin D, and protein.

SEATED SQUEEZES

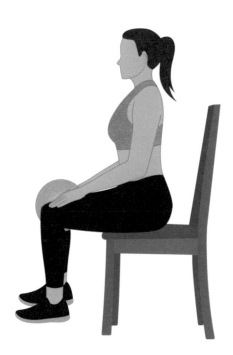

- Sit upright on a chair with your feet flat on the floor.
- Place a cushion or exercise ball between your knees.
- Squeeze the cushion or ball with your knees as hard as you can and hold for three to five seconds.
- Release and relax for a few seconds.
- Repeat 10 to 15 times.

CHAPTER 5: ADVANCED PELVIC FLOOR STRENGTHENING

BAND-ASSISTED LEG LIFTS

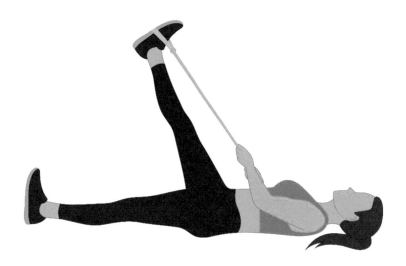

- Lie on your back and loop a resistance band around one foot, holding the ends with your hands for tension.
- Keep the other foot flat on the ground and lift the banded leg straight up towards the ceiling while keeping your pelvis steady.
- Lower it back down slowly.
- Perform 10 to 15 repetitions, then switch legs.

BALL SQUATS

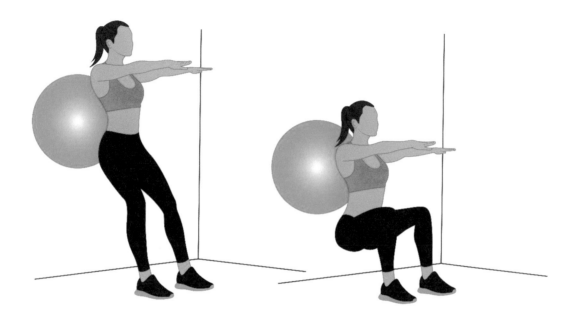

- Stand with your back to a wall with a stability ball placed between the wall and your lower back.
- Spread your feet shoulder-width apart.
- Bend your knees and lower your body into a squat while the ball rolls along your back.
- Lower until your thighs are parallel to the ground, then press back up to the starting position.
- Repeat 10 to 15 times.

PELVIC TILTS WITH STABILITY BALL

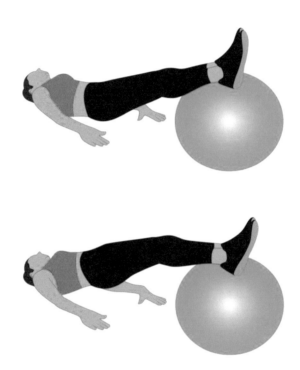

- Lie on your back with your legs resting on top of a stability ball.
- Flatten your back against the floor by tightening your abdominal muscles and tilting your pelvis upwards.
- Hold for a few seconds, then relax back to the starting position.
- Repeat 10 to 15 times.

RESISTANCE BAND SQUATS

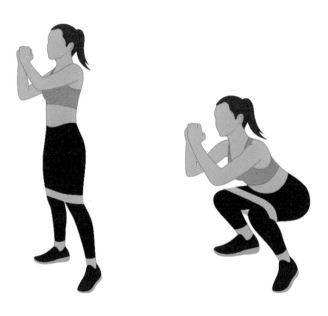

- Stand with feet hip-width apart, stepping on a resistance band.
- Hold the ends of the band at shoulder level.
- Squat down, pushing your hips back and keeping your chest up.
- Return to standing, tightening your glutes as you rise.
- Repeat 10 to 15 times.

It is time to proceed to more advanced techniques for pelvic floor strengthening, designed for those individuals who have already mastered the basic pelvic floor strengthening exercises.

Incorporating Equipment

Quite similar to how we use weights or exercise balls, similar equipments could be incorporated into your pelvic floor exercise routine, which will help in challenging their pelvic floor muscles further, for greater strength and endurance.

- Resistance bands: Quite often used in different exercise routines, resistance bands have the advantage of being cheap and easily procurable, but should also be used with caution, as releasing a resistance band while it is under tension could result in serious injuries. While using a resistance band for the first time, proceed with caution, and do the exercise slowly, till you have familiarised yourself with its usage. Although they are easily stretchable, do not over-stretch it beyond 2.5 times its original length. This could result in accidental breakage, and subsequent injuries. While using a resistance band, that you are standing on an even surface. Banded side steps and leg lifts are the best exercises for your pelvic floor muscles. To do banded side steps, place the resistance band over your thighs or ankles, based on your comfort. Stand with your feet apart, and slowly squat to a half-squat position. Step to your sides, while a resistance should be felt where the band is placed. While stepping, ensure that your knees are pointed outwards, and not inwards. Take 10-15 side steps, and resume the original position. Similarly, to do leg lifts, place the band around your thighs or ankles, and stand with your feet apart. Raise your leg laterally, till you feel the resistance. Do 10 raises each, on both legs.

- Stability Balls: Since pelvic floor muscles play an important role in giving balance and coordination to our body, stability balls could also be incorporated into pelvic floor workouts. Make sure to get a ball that suits your height, and it should be firm, but not too inflated. Ball squats are perfect for enhancing pelvic floor muscles. Choose a stability ball, and place it against a flat surface, ideally a wall. Stand on the other side, so that the ball is placed between the wall and your back. Place your feet at least one foot apart, and let your arms hang loosely by your sides. look straight ahead, and inhale. While exhaling, lower your body straight downwards, till your thighs are parallel to the floor. Now, slowly lift your body, and resume the original position. Do ten reps of the same exercise. You can also do pelvic tilts with a stability ball. Sit on the stability ball, while keeping the back straight. Your feet should be hip-width apart, and your knees should be placed at right angles to the floor. Take a deep inhalation, while rolling the tailbone forwards. When exhaling, roll back, and resume the original position. Repeat 10 times.

- Weights: Although weights are commonly used in strength training, many of us might not be aware of using weights for pelvic floor muscles. Known as Kegel weights or vaginal cones, these are small weights usually made of silicon, which are inserted into the vagina, to strengthen and enhance pelvic floor muscles, usually weakened either by pregnancy, age, or surgical procedures. You can do the regular Kegel exercises with these weights, which impart extra resistance, thus enhancing the muscles.

Exercises to Avoid or Modify for Pelvic Floor Safety

It is indubitable that we all need to stay active for better physical and mental health. However, not all exercises are for everyone. For example, one with a knee injury would stay away from exercises that involve jumping. Similarly, there are exercises that could potentially weaken the pelvic floor muscles, which should be either avoided or modified by those with weakened pelvic floor, or those aiming for enhancing their pelvic floor muscles.

Exercises that put a lot of pressure on abdomen, including crunches, or sit-ups, and heavy impact exercises that require weight lifting or jumping, are few exercises that could weaken the pelvic floor muscles. But does that mean you should stop doing them completely? No! There are modifications you can bring to them, which will make them more pelvic floor-friendly.

For example, while doing exercises like planks and push-ups, make sure to rest your knees on the ground, to perform modified planks and push-ups, which will not impact the pelvic floor muscles. Weight training could also be done, but make sure you are not over-exerting yourself with heavy weights, which might result in bearing down. Weight training while sitting down also helps, and avoid holding your breath while lifting weights. While doing squats, either use a stability ball(described above), or make sure to keep your feet hip-wide apart, and avoid lowering yourself below the knees. Exercises like walking, swimming, yoga, and pilates are also conducive to good pelvic floor health.

Building a Progressive Exercise Routine

To ensure a sustainable and progressive exercise routine, make sure that you listen to your body, by not over exerting yourself. Begin at a slow and comfortable pace, and make slow but steady advancements. Be consistent and regular with your efforts, but take breaks if necessary.

If you are someone who works out regularly, try combining pelvic floor workouts in between regular workouts, thereby reaping more benefits. For instance, while taking a break between your exercise regimen, try doing pelvic squeezes or Kegel exercises. Diaphragmatic breathing is a must, which can be practiced at any time. Let us look at a sample combination of effective pelvic floor exercises.

Here, we are combining two exercises, called heel slides and marches, appropriate for the enhancement of pelvic floor muscles. Heel slides could be done by lying on your back in a comfortable position. Ensure that your knees are bent at right angles. Take a deep inhalation, and exhale through your mouth. While exhaling, slowly slide your right foot away from your body, only till you do not lose control of your core. Hold for two seconds, and bring the foot back to the original position. Repeat on the other foot. Marches are done by lying on your back, and knees at right angles. Slowly lift one leg into the air, and bring it to the tabletop position. Hold for two seconds, and resume the original position. Repeat on the other leg. Combining heel slides and marches, with a set of Kegel exercises in between is a perfect way to create a combined pelvic floor exercise.

CHAPTER 6: PELVIC FLOOR FRIENDLY LIFESTYLE CHANGES

While exercises are crucial for strengthening the pelvic floor, integrating specific lifestyle changes can significantly enhance the benefits of these exercises. Let us explore various adjustments we can make in our daily lives to support and maintain pelvic floor health.

Diet and Hydration

A healthy and balanced approach to life is largely constituted by the two pillars of diet and healthy movement. While exercise is integral to a healthy mind and body, the role of nutrition is not any less.

For optimum health of your pelvic floor muscles, you should ensure that you are including a variety of nutrients like omega fatty acids, and foods rich in Vitamin D in your diet. Natural sources of omega fatty acids include fats fromfish like salmon and mackerel, nuts and seeds like flaxseeds and walnuts, and plants like Brusselssprouts, soybeans, and leafy greens. Foods like egg yolks, cheese, fish, liver, mushrooms, and milk are rich in Vitamin D. It is also important to get enough sunshine as well. If you already have pelvic floor dysfunction, remember to avoid acidic food including acidic fruits, as it could worsen the condition. Instead, consume fruits like bananas or melons, which are less acidic in nature. Remember to keep yourselves hydrated, as optimum levels of hydration are necessary for pelvic floor muscles. Remember to drink at least 2.5-3 litres of water a day, depending on your levels of activity, and other factors like temperature. Keeping yourself hydrated is key in digestion, and prevents constipation and other disorders.

Weight Management and Its Impact on Pelvic Health

How is our weight related to pelvic health? The link is quite easy to understand. A person with more body weight will experience greater pressure on their pelvic floor. The body fat exerts pressure on the pelvic organs including the bladder and bowels, thus resulting in difficulties in the movement of urine or fecal matter. Research shows that individuals with greater BMI are more prone to contracting urinary incontinence, as opposed to others(Khullar et al., 2013).

Although there are no shortcuts to lose weight, a balanced approach will get you to your goals, in a sustainable manner. Instead of going through fad diets and depriving yourself, the focus should fall on consuming a balanced and nutritious diet, along with consistent exercise routine. This is especially important for the senior population, as nutritionally restrictive diets could seriously tamper with your health.

Posture and Ergonomics to Support Pelvic Floor Muscles

As mentioned in the earlier chapters, poor posture is one of the most common factors for weakened pelvic floor muscles. Most of us slouch while standing or walking, which is detrimental to the health of pelvic floor muscles. Ensure that while standing or walking, the weight of your body is resting on the balls of your feet, and not on the heels or the toes. The shoulders should be slightly pulled backwards. While sitting, do not cross your legs, but rest them comfortably on the floor. Your shoulders should be relaxed, but the back should be straight, or if needed, you can use a support like a cushion. If your job requires you to sit for longer periods, do not forget to stretch and walk once in a while.

Some ergonomic adjustments could be brought into your daily routine. For example, if you spend considerable time working on a computer, ensure to keep a back support, and your shoulders relaxed. Make sure that your chair is sturdy but comfortable, and should follow your spine's natural curve. Take breaks in between to stretch yourself, or go for a short walk.

Managing Constipation and Proper Toilet Habits

Constipation is a serious condition that affects the pelvic floor muscles, which might become loose as a result of constant straining. There are many factors which lead to constipation, including improper diet, lack of hydration, and lack of physical activity. In order to ensure the prevention of constipation, one should include a lot of fiber in your diatom including wholegrain, fresh vegetables, and fruits. Keep yourself hydrated, and make sure to indulge in some kind of physical activity every day. Set aside some time for your toilet break, which is helpful in preventing constipation.

While sitting on the toilet, use a foot support to ensure that your knees are higher than your hips, which also prevents slouching. Slightly lean forward, and place your elbows on the knees. Relax, and do proper breathing.

Reducing Strain During Daily Activities

Many of the daily activities, like lifting, bad posture, and staining, could be detrimental to the health of your pelvic muscles. Ensure to keep your feet together, and maintain a good posture while lifting. Do not hold your breath, while it is also advised to try pelvic muscle contractions while lifting, which prevents muscle damage. Smoking exacerbates the weakening of pelvic floor muscle, as it triggers respiratory ailments. While sneezing, coughing, or laughing, we unconsciously exert pressure on the pelvic floor. An easy alternative to prevent this, is by slightly turning your head to the side while on such occasions, which lessens the strain on the perineum. Similarly, train yourself to contact the pelvic muscles during coughing or sneezing, which eventually becomes a habit.

Stress Management and Its Role in Pelvic Floor Health

Did you know that there is a link between stress and pelvic floor dysfunction? Although experiencing stress is part of the experience of life, chronic stress, or stress that lasts over a period of time, could have unfavorable effects on our general health. Stress hormones such as epinephrine and norepinephrine increase the blood flow, and cause the muscles to tense, forcing them to remain in this state over a long time. This adversely impacts the muscles, and results in their dysfunction. To prevent this, we need to take adequate steps to address our stress.

To maneuverthrough stress, one needs to acknowledge it first. Techniques like meditation, yoga, and self-reflection through journaling are steps that might help you recover from chronic stress. Connecting with others is important to alleviate stress. You could join support groups or clubs to meet people with similar interests, or participate in activities like volunteering. Physical activity is unavoidable, as the dopamine released through physical activity, also known as the happy hormone, plays a key role in relaxation.

CHAPTER 7: OVERCOMING COMMON CHALLENGES

Embarking on a journey to improve pelvic floor health can be filled with ups and downs. Let us look at some common challenges and setbacks that we may face, and strategies for overcoming them and progressing towards our goal.

Dealing with Setbacks and Lack of Progress

While exercising to build muscles, one might come across a situation where the initial progress comes to a stupor. Although this could occur at any time, normally it is seen after 1-2 months of starting a routine. This could be read as a demotivating sign by many people, as discernible progress is definitely motivating. However, this phenomenon, also known as hitting a plateau, is quite common in muscle building exercises.

To prevent yourself from getting demotivated, switch your workouts niece in while, and introduce variety in your regime, either by changing the warm-up routine, or going for a swim or a walk instead. Try to be consistent in recording the slightest improvements, either by using an app or a simple journal. Plateauing could also be a sign for amping up the intensity of your routine, which should be introduced slowly, but deliberately. If required, you could also seek support from a trainer or a healthcare professional.

Managing Discomfort During Exercises

While it is quite normal to experience some kind of discomfort, especially dung the initial phase of your muscle training, if the pain gets too uncomfortable, it is a sign that you are overexerting yourself, or the techniques are wrong. Usually, the soreness that one feels after exercise, results from a muscle group getting exposed to training after a while. It usually goes away after a while, but the bad pain usually results from injury or bad technique, and it gets worse.

If you experience prolonged discomfort while exercising, it is a sign to modify your exercise regimen. You could try reducing the intensity or duration of the workout, and seek the help of an expert to analyse if your technique or posture is wrong.

Adjusting Exercises for Other Health Issues

Many elderly people suffer from weak knees, joints, or arthritis, which could make exercising difficult. However, if taken necessary precautions, exercising could not only be fun, but also could make your joint pain better! First and foremost, keep your exercises low-impact. If necessary, you could do modified versions of regular exercises. For example, for those with knee pain, doing chair squats or using a stability ball could be useful. Before exercising, either use a warm towel to press on the muscles or take a warm shower, which will help heal sore muscles. Additionally, you could also use ice packs after the exercise, especially if you have swollen joints.

If you have had a pelvic floor exercise, seek the advice of your doctor on when you could restart the exercise regimen. In most cases a period of 3-6 weeks is recommended before even starting lighter exercises like walking or pelvic squeezes. Remember to start gently and support the lower abdomen area during the initial phase. It is better to seek the support of a qualified trainer while restarting your routine.

Addressing Psychological Barriers

It is seldom that conversations around pelvic floor health and issues such as incontinence happen in the public space. As a result, many of us find it difficult to open up about such topics, even to a medical practitioner. However, there are many people who share similar issues, and joining in support groups or societies that encourage discussions on pelvic floor health is a great step to start our journey. Additionally, mindfulness techniques could be used to combat negative thoughts and anxiety related to pelvic floor issues, fostering a more positive and proactive approach to pelvic health.

Finding the Right Professional Help

Manoeuvring through an exercise regimen could be difficult for the elder population, especially if they are introduced to it for the first time. While it is normal for you to experience sore muscles especially in the initial stages of the routine, do not hesitate to seek professional help if the pain persists, or of the pain is causing discomfort which affects the quality of your life.

However, which expert should you see? In case of post-operative issues or post-natal issues, remember to put your doctors first, which, depending on the type of surgery, could be urologists or gynecologists. There are specialist physiotherapists who specialize in pelvic floor issues who could provide solutions for pelvic pain and general discomfort. If you experience painful intercourse or sexual issues such as erectile dysfunction, a sexologist should be your first point of reference. Physiotherapists can also be sought if you are seeking advice to improve your posture.

Once you have made an appointment, remember to write down the details correctly, so that you can be completely transparent with them. There is no absolute need for embarrassment, as they are experts who have been trained to deal with similar cases every day.

CHAPTER 8: INTEGRATING PELVIC FLOOR HEALTH INTO DAILY LIFE

Achieving and maintaining a healthy pelvic floor goes beyond isolated exercises. This chapter focuses on how to seamlessly integrate pelvic floor health practices into daily life, ensuring sustainable habits that support long-term well-being

Tips for Incorporating Pelvic Floor Exercises into Everyday Activities

In addition to setting a fixed routine for exercise, pelvic floor exercises could be incorporated into your daily activities like walking, sitting, or standing. Many of us suffer from weak pelvic muscles due to improper posture. For example, while walking, one should place their heels on the floor first, while the rest of the foot should follow. While walking, breathe normally, while simultaneously doing pelvic squeezes.

Similarly, while standing, ensure that your weight is supported uniformly by the two legs, and you have placed your feet slightly apart. Make sure your spine is straight, with a slight inward bend at the lower back.

If your job demands you to sit for longer periods of time, it is crucial to correct your sitting posture. While your weight should ideally be distributed equally on your two sit bones, your feet should be hip-wide apart. Never slouch, or droop your head, but your crown should be pointed towards the ceiling. If required, use a back support. Take breaks in between to stretch or walk.

In all three cases, practice diaphragmatic breathing.

While lifting weights or small kids, remember to keep your feet together, and maintain good posture. Exhale thoroughly while lifting, and do pelvic squeezes along with the exhalation.

Using Mindfulness and Stress Reduction to Support Pelvic Health

We had explored the concept of mindfulness in one of the previous chapters. The quality of mindfulness is essential when it comes to improving focus and alleviating stress. Pelvic dysfunction and allied disorders could be sources of embarrassment and discomfort to many, thus increasing their stress levels. However, it high stress levels only exacerbates our physical and mental health, thus affecting the quality of life.

However, by being mindful and practicing stress reduction techniques such as meditation and yoga, we can reduce stress to a considerable extent. Let us look at a sample mindfulness exercise.

One of the most effective and simple mindfulness exercises is called a body scan. To do this exercise, sit or lie down in a comfortable position. Focus your attention on yourself, and breathe deeply. Slowly begin from your toes. Focus your attention on your toes, and listen to your body. Watch out for any symptoms of pain or discomfort. Slowly, shift the attention to the legs, and continue the process till the entire body is scanned.

This helps in relaxing, as well as improving our general focus.

Lifestyle Modifications for Optimal Pelvic Floor Health

The two pillars of a healthy body and mind are optimal nutrition and proper physical activity. These are essential elements when it comes to maintaining a healthy weight and preventing many health conditions.

Instead of jumping on the bandwagon of fad diets, it is vital to follow a nutritious, and balanced diet. As we age, muscles tend to get weaker, as they are exposed to regular wear and tear. Therefore, it is important to include nutrients such as protein, Vitamin D, Calcium, Magnesium, and healthy fats in your diet. Carbohydrates are an important source of energy; however, ensure that your source of carbohydrates includes unrefined and unprocessed whole grains and cereals. It is best to avoid the consumption of processed foods, sugar, and alcohol and limit the intake of caffeine.

Regular physical activity is unavoidable, as it is not only vital for the health of muscles and bones, but also promotes good mental health.

Sexual Health and Pelvic Floor Well-being

Sexual health and pelvic floor well-being are related concepts, as explained in the previous chapters. However, sexual issues are also less discussed, owing to them being a taboo in our society.

In men, a weak pelvic floor could result in premature ejaculation and erectile dysfunction, while in women, it could manifest in the form of painful intercourse. As they could potentially affect the quality of your lives, it is vital that partners should have open discussions on how they affect sexual health, fostering understanding and mutual support.

Enjoyable sex is still possible in such cases, which could be fostered through mutual support. Open communication is the first step, which can allow you to discover positions that are comfortable for both parties. The use of lubricant and buffer rings can reduce penetrative pain and discomfort to a considerable degree. You could revitalize your sexual life by trying new techniques and positions and through using sex toys.

Preparing for Changes in Pelvic Floor Health Over Time

As we age, there will arise multiple factors which could complicate your pelvic floor health, including menopause in women, and andropause in men. These phases are characterized by the lowering of sex hormones and the resultant health conditions that affect pelvic floor health. Pelvic organ prolapse and pelvic dysfunction are found in many people who go through this phase.

By preparing for such changes, one can avoid much pain and discomfort. By making the right lifestyle choices, doing regular check-ups, and staying informed about pelvic health, one can enjoy their retired lives in perfect peace and happiness.

CHAPTER 9: SPECIAL CONSIDERATIONS FOR MEN

While pelvic floor health is often associated with women, particularly in the context of pregnancy and childbirth, it's equally important for men. Let us look at some unique aspects of male pelvic floor health, such as conditions specific to men, exercises tailored for male anatomy, and strategies for integrating pelvic floor health into daily life.

Understanding Male Pelvic Floor Health

Balls

Weakened pelvic floor muscles in men could potentially result in many major health conditions. When it comes to sexual health, erectile dysfunction, and hard flaccid syndrome, which affect sexual performance. Erectile dysfunction is characterized by the condition when an individual experiences difficulty in forming and maintaining an erection of their penis. Hard flaccid syndrome, on the other hand, could be identified by multiple symptoms including painful ejaculation, shortening of the penis, or changes in sensation, which is caused by weakening of pelvic muscles. Issues in incontinence such as PMD or post-micturition dribble and incontinence developed after surgical procedures are a few other issues that affect men, which could be corrected through a consistent pelvic floor routine.

Tailored Exercises for Men

Exercises for the pelvic floor, be it basic or advanced exercises, require to be performed consistently, while being mindful of the right technique. We have discussed the right way of doing Kegel exercises in the earlier chapters. How can we ensure that a man is doing Kegel in the right form? The first step is to ensure that your pelvic muscles are in action, and not your abdominal muscles. The muscles that you contract while stopping urination are your pelvic muscles.

Contract the pelvic muscles slowly, while you might be able to feel a sensation similar to lifting. Hold it for five to ten seconds, but continue breathing normally. Release, and relax. There is no fixed time when you should do this, in fact, you could do this during any time of the day, even while traveling, exercising, at office, or even while watching TV.

Bridges and squats with stability balls are other exercises that you can do.

Addressing Male-Specific Concerns: Issues and Lifestyle Changes

Some of the most common male-specific concerns related to the pelvic floor include erectile dysfunction, incontinence, and post-operative discomfort. Kegel exercises make much positive difference when it comes to erectile dysfunction. Here is a Kegel exercise with a difference, meant for corrective erectile dysfunction.

Lie on your back comfortably, with your hands resting on the sides, and knees bent at right angles. Breathe comfortably. Now try to withdraw your penis inwards, holding it for five seconds. Release, and relax. Repeat five times.

Remember to keep yourself hydrated, eat a diet rich in omega fatty acids and magnesium, and limit your intake of alcohol, sugar, and processed foods. Smoking is one of the most dangerous habits that exacerbate the condition, and hence should be avoided at all costs.

Regular kegels and squats are advised for incontinence, however, when it comes to post-operative incontinence, make sure to seek the advice of your doctor when and how to resume your exercise regimen. Foods that improve the health of the urinary tract, for example, whole grains, lean protein, and fruits such as bananas, pears, and vegetables should be more included in the diet.

Overcoming Barriers to Pelvic Floor Health in Men

With the right information and approach, men can overcome common conditions affecting their pelvic floor, enhancing their health and life satisfaction. Destigmatizing pelvic floor conditions is necessary to create an atmosphere where men can talk openly about their health concerns. The first step towards that is to understand that pelvic floor disorders are common, and are like any other health issue, for which necessary help must be sought. Talk to health practitioners, or be a part of support groups and organizations where you can be a part of wider conversations on the topic. For more insight into such groups, see the next chapter.

CHAPTER 10: MOVING FORWARD WITH CONFIDENCE

As we conclude our journey through understanding and improving pelvic floor health, this chapter focuses on empowering readers to continue their progress with confidence. It outlines how to set realistic goals, recognize when to seek professional help, and embrace pelvic health as a lifelong commitment

Setting Realistic Goals and Tracking Progress

We hear a lot about setting realistic goals when it comes to starting an exercise routine. Why are they important? For every work that we do, to ensure the progress is sustainable and continuous, we need to set defined and clear goals. This will help us stick to the regimen, and stay motivated.

But what are realistic goals? To make the process easier, let us ask ourselves certain questions. Why am I doing this? How much time do I have? What is my major goal? How can I split my major goal into smaller parts, each allotted a specific time frame? These questions will guide you through setting definable, precise, and realistic goals for yourself. Remember to be non-judgmental and honest with yourself while setting the goals.

Having set the goals, use a fitness tracker app or an exercise journal to measure your progress. Note down the particularities of your exercise regimen, external measurements like your weight, and even related factors like your nutrition and hydration.

Acknowledging and celebrating improvements, no matter how small, is as important as abiding by your goals, to maintain motivation and commitment to health. Once you have reached your smaller sub-goals, treat yourself to a self-care day, or celebrate by gifting yourself something.

Embracing Pelvic Health as a Key Component of Senior Wellness

Contrary to popular misconceptions, pelvic floor health is not only related to continence, but it has an overall impact on our general wellness. It affects multiple factors like our balance and posture, bowel and urinary movement, and sexual wellness. Thus, taking care of pelvic floor wellness adds a holistic aspect to our wellness and health nourishment.

This is particularly important as we age, since weakened pelvic floor muscles poses greater health risks during the later years of our lives. You might have heard many old people complaining about how their lives have become dependent on others, and how old age poses serious threats to one's self-efficacy and independence. However, by taking proper care of our pelvic floor muscles, we can prevent many such psychological and physical issues. By spending some time on pelvic floor enhancement regularly, we are making a lifelong commitment to better emotional and physical wellness. Depending on your activity levels, medical condition, and age, your pelvic floor work our regimen could be customized, through incorporating basic to advanced exercises, depending on your requirements.

Building a Support Network and Staying Updated

Exercise tends to get boring when it is a lonely affair, and it is a prominent reason why many get demotivated soon. Think about a situation where one is a part of a group of many like-minded individuals, who share similar goals and insights, who motivate each other. It will undoubtedly create a space conducive to growth and sustainability.

By joining classes and support groups, you can find such spaces where mutual interactions and encouragement are possible. Even if physical interaction is not possible, there are many virtual groups available online, where one can connect with people from different parts of the world. International Pelvic Pain Society, Pelvic Pain Support Network, Pelvic Floor Dysfunction Support Group, and Sisters for Pelvic Health are some of the online support groups for pelvic health.

It is also a good idea to take the initiative yourselves, by hosting a meeting for your friends and family, where you could talk about the benefits of a pelvic floor routine, thus bringing more people to the benefits of pelvic floor enhancement.

Staying updated is as important as sticking to an exercise regime. Medical science and health sector are growing everyday, with the latest inventions and research making groundbreaking changes. By staying abreast of the latest news on pelvic floor health, we are not only updating ourselves, but also reaping the benefits of the latest science and technology. For example, here is a resource list of some of the books, journals, and websites that provide the latest information on the topic.

Books- HOPE For Your Pelvic Floor by Claire Catherine Sparrow, Healing Pelvic Pain By Amy Stein, A Headache in the Pelvis by David Stein, Pelvic Floor Essentials By Sue Croft, and A Woman's Guide to Pelvic Health by Elizabeth Houser and Stephanie Hahn.

Journals- Journal of Women's & Pelvic Health Physical Therapy, Pelviperineology: A Multidisciplinary Pelvic Floor Journal, and International Urogynecology Journal.

Websites- Your Pelvic Floor(https://www.yourpelvicfloor.org), POGP(https://thepogp.co.uk/), Pelvic Floor First(https://www.pelvicfloorfirst.org.au), Pelvic Health Physio(https://www.pelvichealth-physio.com), and Pelvic Health Solutions(https://pelvichealthsolutions.ca)

Improving and maintaining pelvic floor health is a rewarding journey that enhances the quality of life and overall well-being. By setting realistic goals, seeking professional guidance when necessary, and viewing pelvic health as a lifelong commitment, we can move forward with confidence.

CONCLUSION

We hope you have not only gained a deeper understanding of your pelvic floor, but also feel equipped and motivated to incorporate these exercises into your routine.

Although conversations on general wellness and psychological health are encouraged and are practiced widely, pelvic floor wellness and associated mental and physical implications are not so widely discussed. We hope this book will serve as an impetus to kindle more such conversations, as well as spark a collective interest in care for pelvic health.

It is never too late to start focusing on your pelvic health. As this book has demonstrated, small but collected and consistent steps are what matters in this journey. If you have found this book helpful, kindly leave a positive review, which will motivate us to write more on such topics.

REFERENCES

Batmani, S., Jalali, R., Mohammadi, M., & Bokaee, S. (2021). Prevalence and Factors Related to Urinary Incontinence in Older Adults Women Worldwide: A Comprehensive Systematic Review and Meta-Analysis of Observational Studies. *BMC Geriatrics (Online)*, *21*(1).

Callewaert, G., Albersen, M., Janssen, K., Damaser, Van Mieghem, T., Van Der Vaart, C., & Deprest, J. (2015). The Impact of Vaginal Delivery on Pelvic Floor Function – Delivery as a Time Point for Secondary Prevention. *BJOG: An International Journal of Obstetrics and Gynaecology*, *123*(5), 678–681.

Forsgren, C., Amato, M., & Johannesson, U. (2022). Effects of Hysterectomy on Pelvic Floor Function and Sexual Function—A Prospective Cohort Study. *Acta Obstetricia Et Gynecologica Scandinavica*, *101*(10), 1048–1056.

Hagen, S, et al. (2014). Individualised Pelvic Floor Muscle Training in Women with Pelvic Organ Prolapse (POPPY): A Multicentre Randomised Controlled Trial. *The Lancet*, *383*(9919), 796–806.

Khullar, V, et al. (2013). The Relationship Between BMI and Urinary Incontinence Subgroups: Results from EpiLUTS. *Neurourology and Urodynamics*, *33*(4), 392–399.

25553464R00033